One Light

One Light

by Dana Wildsmith

Texas Review Press • Huntsville, Texas

Requests for permission to acknowledge material from this work should be sent to: Permissions, Texas Review Press, Sam Houston State University, Huntsville, TX 77341-2146

Library of Congress Cataloging-in-Publication Data can be found at www.loc.gov.

For Don

And for Will Balk and Pauletta Hansel, who know

Contents

One Light

A single light can lead you home. One light
is all you need to break the back of night
when darkness seems to weigh more than it has
on all the nights before, and nothing's as
it was. Bit by bit, the lighter shades
of night you used to trust have faded as
you stopped believing in relief . The dark
goes on forever, and begins right where you are.

But when your eyes can't guide your steps, you learn
to trust your heart instead. You rise and turn
toward where you need to go, and in the dark
you think you see a glimmer like a star
that wasn't there until you headed home
through darkness, trusting that a light would come.

Saving

Sometimes it is the artist's task to find out how much music you can still make with what you have left.

—Itzhak Perlman

How it Happened

It was one of those February nights
that give us of the deep South an excuse
to start a fire in the mostly unused
fireplace, a clear night as stern as marble,
not even a far cloud to snug the stars
like a bunting.

           The coziest way to be
on such a night is angled toward heat,
feet wide apart on the hearth, elbows and
open book on the mantle, a slow draft
of warm air hilling over the snoring
dog and upward under a floor-length
nightgown.

           It was my dog who was sleeping
on beige carpeting that particular evening,
and my bare legs which were toasting under
a flannel gown ballooned with heated air.
I was reading, and the room was quiet,
except for the dog's easy huffing breaths,
except for the hiss of gas

                  and the pop
of sparks from gas-fired ceramic logs.
I had just turned fourteen, well old enough
to know that the calm of a close blond room
can't last. If the phone had rung then, or if
my mother had had reason to come in,
I would have been annoyed,

                  yet not surprised.

But no one bothered me. The flames grew high
as canna lilies. I leaned more forward
as I read, my muscles stunned with comfort.
Looking down toward the bottom of the next
page, I saw a motion out of context,
a bright fleck

      like a fire flea hopping
to the hem of my gown and burrowing in,
as fleas will. That's what I saw: the quick arc
of a small bug's jump. And then, as if warp
and weft were branchings of nerves, as if
the cloth of my gown were irritated skin,
a splotch of red

        splashed upward from my hem.
Flames petaled like gladiolas toward my hands,
hands trying to do the mind's business
and the mind like flame consuming itself.
Not a sound came from me and no sounds
reached me to interrupt the solemn
proceedings involving me

        as clear nights
involve stars, as sleep involves dreams. Despite
however long it may have seemed that I
stood mesmerized within that caul, only
a flicker of time had passed, a moment,
one breath-hold. Just time enough for mama
halfway through her bath

        to wash one arm from
shoulder to hand, for our gas meter to
click to the next higher number, one car
to whizz past our house, and for my dachshund's

howling to bring me around to a panic
that reeled me out of the room. My hip
hit the dining room table,

          and I put
out my hand for balance, but never felt
my left hand touch wood, even when it did.
That whole left side was forfeit, given
as fuel, leaving just my voice as residue.
Such as it was, my voice, remnant of
what had been me,

          worked well enough to call
my mama from her bath. She grabbed wet towels
and swaddled me. As soon as the fire was out,
the dining room reappeared. I found
myself on the floor beside the table.
I could see my mama's legs, the metal
chair legs,

         the wood floor. I could see my hands.
My hands were raisins, powdery old ones
withered to grey pebbles. They were charcoal,
hard, and wrapped in clear plastic. Splintered
posts with a whitish hang of something crumpled.
Two mildewed gloves. Fungus on a twigged stump.
Mold.

   I held my hands out in front of me
and studied them: two raku pieces
fresh from the kiln. The house was dead quiet,
mama watching me for signs of shock, daddy
watching for the ambulance, and me-
as calm as ever I remember being.
My hands did not hurt.

There was no pain.
I tell you, fire is not an agonizing
sizzle. It is the grim pull of muscled
hands (climber's hands, potter's hands) tugging
deadened skin from bone while you watch. It is
twilight sleep. No one ever believes this.
Years later,

and years after these healed hands
have come back to me like a vow, I can
no more now than I could then convince
my sympathetic listeners that the pain
they think I felt while I was burning
is not the hurt that haunts me. How can I tell them
they are wrong?

They who have never known
the numbness of destruction would be
discomfited to hear that years after these
hands have rooted back to me like a born child,
I still would dress myself in lengths of flame
before I would again face that moment
after burning when I saw the marbled ruin
of my hands.

(This is an old argument.
Remember, you have only what I
tell you. You are in a garden, blind,
and I have been making small pale flowers
out of words.)

Keeping Watch

Only when I had a daughter of
my own and not until her fourteenth year
did I begin to watch for signs of fire,
or meteors, or fevers—any spark
that might blaze up and take her down.
I hadn't known this fear lay banked in me.
When Mama saved me for my fifteenth year
by feeding her own hands into that fire
unmaking me, she interfered with fate,
but debt deferred is yet a debt. The span
I should have lived, transferred to my own child,
and fire my mama thought she'd doused
flared out of reason's reach the year
my daughter aged into my destiny.

After Midnight

As soon as I didn't die, the surgeon
who'd been paged from his basement poker game
gave my parents the odds: *if she makes it
through the night, she'll lose both hands,
if not her whole left arm.*

                      Then he cut off my rings,
one numb tug and then another to save
my hands, not the rings, gambling on
my dying hands as not yet dead, playing
against my odds.

Emergency Room

The neutral air has neutral hands that lift
and roll and—on my count—lay me down.
Fingers insinuate through mist to strip
and survey me. The hallways mumble and frown.
One man's eyes lack the grace to pretend; I wish
he had the grace to leave. Words priss around
my gurney, conferring. Machines sidle in
like auditors. Liquid sleep slides down
its tubular tributary. *Lullay, lully,*
it croons. This is not my concern. *Hush now.*

Hospital Days

Being tubbed and scrubbed of fourteen years
of flesh now charred to hard crusts, being wound
with fresh gauze from feet to neck, being doused
with icy silver nitrate, my day nurse
razzed and joked while she debrided me--

                                    Come on,
it ain't so bad as that. We're almost done.
Then she'd step outside to cry, because pity
kills. The rest of the day, she'd marinate me,
ladling from a silver bowl the silver nitrate
to cleanse my arms and back. All day

                        I swam
in a cold black sea that ebbed through the night
as the gauze dried and stuck to my burns skin-tight.
Every morning, my nurse would rip it off.
That felt exactly as you'd think it might.
And yet--

                what I remember, too, are hot dogs
from the deli downstairs for lunch, a friend
who brought her guitar and sang with me
to keep my lungs strong—*Up, up with people,*
They're best kinda folks I know.

                        Then Chloe,
my nurse, would prop me with pillows and zoom me
along every ward except maternity;
those new mothers didn't need to see me.
Once Chloe secreted us through a door
in a basement storeroom,

                    a low doorway
that led to a tunnel to the river
where narrow slabs of stone had been beds for
our wounded soldiers during the war. She said
they lay in that dark and echoing damp
waiting for death or for deliverance.

                              Mama
brought the best of the world to me
when she came to relieve Chloe at three:
a milk shake, a book projector I worked
with my toe, a thick stack of cards to read,
my dog smuggled in,
                         and Mama, herself.

Once she let a man in to pray for me,
but he declaimed my burns as the wages
of my sins and reached for me. Mama lied
to save me from him:

             We're not allowed to touch her
because of germs, as she shooed him out the door
with the grace only southern women own,
and we both went back to reading the books
we'd talk about later, she said,

                  when I was home.

Who Stays

Who, asked night air, hazy with hall light,
who stays with her?
I, said Mother, forsaking the father.
I stay with her.

Who, asked the father patting the bedclothes,
who stays with me?
We, said the children, biting their lips.
We stay with you.

Who, asked the children when no one could hear,
who stays with us?
I, said the home place, closing one door.
I stay with you.

Who, asked the home place shifting its footings,
who stays with me?
I, begged the burned child alone with the night.
I'll stay with you.

What You Need

A touch that no one is required to give.
A touch that's more than maintenance, more
than being tended with the economy
of touch appropriate to skinlessness.
They love me best who touch me least.
This is how it feels to be uncherished,
this parameter between what's necessary
and what is needed. Now I understand.
If healing comes, it comes by way of my will,
not their hands.

The Night Nurse

She worked the ER, eleven to seven.
I don't remember the first time she came
to my room before her shift began,
or know how she'd heard I lay there awake
after the hall lights

                    were dimmed for the night.
I do remember the grey congestion
of hospital air, and how chimney smoke
wriggled through air vents, beckoning me.
My narrow bed went rigid with watching,
and my muscles gathered

                    to mournful knots
no one could touch, or ease. Surely, she knew
how untouchable I was, but she'd lean in
until I saw only her rayoned hip
spooning toward her waist, and the blunt dip
of her elbow

           as she massaged my temples,
one of the few strips of skin left to me.
Each night, sleep would remember my face
as I inclined toward the night nurse's hands.
The night blew out its held breath. My bed
gently rocked.

Kinesis

After the fathomless nights of insult,
when pain's debates had droned to a tedium,
I woke to the unshackling notion
that healing can be provoked. I began
to tinker with limits, keeping this to myself,
but visualizing my skin growing back
until hope hummed through my veins
like blood from a clean wound:--
bright and clear and useful.

Intentional Wounds

I had healed enough to be wounded again,
so they scheduled a flaying for Tuesday.
One lone island of unburned skin the shape
of Cuba along my right thigh remained
amid an expanse of black scabs, so Tuesday
my surgeon would harvest this virgin field,
rolling it with a cheese-slicer of sorts,
laying that cellular sod on my arms
and packing his plantings with gauze to shield
his precarious crop and save my hide.

But a body's not meant for skinning
and flesh is not nerveless soil.
I woke to the pain my shocked nerves
had spared me while I was burning.
I woke, and saw nothing
but pain's flaming face looming over me.
Who knew a person could literally see red?

Waking

I woke from drugged sleep to a scald of air,
muted by insult so grievous no words,
no cries, no moans could sound the depth of hurt
that even now I cannot find words for,
except to tell it plain:

                     I was fourteen.

My thighs had been pared like fruit while I slept,
sliced like cheese, and the flood of my blood left
to dry to a rind where they took the skin.
I woke inside my nerve endings--
the only possible explanation for
the blood-colored field that blotted out
my bed, my parents, my doctor.
I saw only red. The mind craves reason,

                     and nothing's reasonable
about skinning a child. My mind took away words
and gave me a color instead, a color that screams,
that furies, that means what it says.

                         Red.

Pain

Pain's the music of process, and it's jazz,
don't you know? Skittery. Can't pin it down.
You wanna find the root and ride it out,
but pain's slick, goes flat for a beat—I've got this.
No, you don't. Pain shifts and bends. Nothing
you can do but forget what you knew. Listen,
there's danger lurkin', 'cause resistance
ain't workin'. You gotta grab it like you want it.
When pain can't shake you, it'll syncopate.
Feel the beat? It's yours now. You own it. Take
the rhythm and run.

Fool Me Once

My surgeon had the hands of a pianist--
strong from use, but he could use them gently
to give my toes a friendly squeeze, or to rest
his hand warmly across my forehead as
his soft bass rumbled of donor skin and grafts
to Mama and Daddy, over my head. I heard,
but didn't listen. His hand smoothed back my hair.
To sleep was all that was required of me,
to sleep and wake, but not quite wake, when
a night-shift aide transferred me to a gurney
and tucked me in with heated sheets to journey
with Mama as far as the O.R.'s outer doors.
 In there, a giant hammer hung on the wall. *See?*
My surgeon grinned. *Anesthesia!*
Then came my second sleep, more profound
and dreamless until he called my name, loud,
then louder: *Dana. Dana? Come on back.*
But there was no coming back. His bloodied hands
had stripped me of belief in easy fixes.
If I could wake to agony like this,
what else? *You did just fine,* he said, and smiled.
It's over now. All done. All done.

                              Liar.

The Languages of Healing

Don't expect pity because you itch.
Oh, this is wonderful, they'll say.
You're healing! Now really, which
is worse, a little itching or pain?

They may as well ask which is worse:
aphasia or dyslexia?
Healing speaks two languages:
the first is pain, which has no words;

the second is itch—just when you think
you've found the root, it flits. Not worse
nor less than pain, itch is
the new translation of misery.

Hey Andy

Hey Andy, betcha never reckoned on
poison ivy when you slid down that tree
in shorts and no shirt, your arms and legs wound
around the trunk for a slicker slide. Me?
I sure never reckoned on fire's quick climb
up my own trunk. When our old skins sloughed off
and new skin came in about the same time,
our mothers got us together to scratch.

Obviously, I've never forgotten
the comfort of shared disfigurement.

Some of Us

Some of us wait for winter.
We are the lucky ones
who kept our faces.
We wait for cold's excuse
to sleeve our scarred arms
and slip mittens over
what's left of our fingers.
Winter brings the benevolence
of sweaters with their refuge
spun out of wool.
Being bundled makes all of us
bulkily similar,
and sameness clings like frost,
so winter's dead world
seems to some of us
fair exchange for the right
to blend in for a while.

On My Other Hand

On my other hand
the skin piles up on itself
in soft pleats
the way a nylon slip
bunches to my thigh
on cold, dry mornings.

This is the hand
that almost died,
sampled by fire,
but snatched back
from death into
instant old age.

Now when I dress
each morning,
a crinkled crone's hand
lifts past my face,
waving to me
from my other hand's future.

My Invisible Scars

Movie theaters.
Elevators.
Lit cigarettes.
Smoke.

That's it.

None of these fears, of course,
has any relation to how I was burned,
at home, in my living room.
There were no smokers in my family,
and no smoke after the flames went out.

But fear claims its own logic.
Fireplaces, gas, and open flames
had had their way with me, so in walked
four new fears of what else might happen.

I can see them now.

The Hardest Part

The hardest part was leaving. April had
gone on without me and the south was well
into Spring.

Everywhere were drifts of azaleas,
pink ones, as pink as I was. The dogwoods
were mottled halfway from flower to leaf.
Magnolia leaves littered the parks like

the curls of my dead skin that flaked away
as I left the hospital. I was molting,
fourteen years peeling off like a snake's skin.

I was as irresistible to people's stares
as the little shoots of Sensitive Fern
you can't help but touch to watch the leaves
close in on themselves.

Shelter Log

Decades later when I gave hiking a try,
I found the only way to train to hike
the A.T. is to hike it. There's nothing like it--
a walking trail from Maine to Georgia that climbs
and dips and switches back on itself and entices
its hikers eternally onward for two thousand miles,
for six months, despite rain and shelter mice
and giardia and bears and blisters. Why
would we do this? The shelter logs tell why:
Today I saw the bear and her cubs I've
been hearing about. Sweet .Hey, hikers, I'm
leaving some fuel I don't need, but you might.
Full moon tomorrow, folks. Bright sky tonight.
Someone tell Shadow I apologize.
Long, steep ascent ahead, but the trail guide
makes it sound worse than it is, no lie.
You can do it. See you on the other side.

Those first few weeks after I was burned
I wasn't allowed any visitors,
so Mama taped a ledger to my door
for friends to sign their names, or leave notes
for me to see later, when I'd made it over
that first long haul. *Hi from Teenie Cowart!*
Raymond and Ronald- we'll see you later.
Gave blood for you--O.H. Zipperer.
Your Trinity MYF group—we're here!
We miss you.

When we left the hospital,
Mama stashed the paper away until
it came time to pass it on to me

along with other proofs of my life,
against the inevitable day she
could no longer vouch for me herself..
Torn along its edges now, I store it
with my birth certificate as the words
that spoke me into being at my birth
and my rebirth.

What Saved Me

I was eight years old, helping Grandmother
ready her rental house between tenants.
We sang Cokesbury hymns while we cleaned and
cleared the kitchen. The white enamel sink
stayed cool despite a wall of tall windows
open to Florida's July inferno,
so I leaned both elbows on its coolness
and sang with Grandmother on the chorus,
Out of the ivory palaces....

Here, I thought. This sink is white as ivory,
and those magnolias out back are palace guards
for Grandmother--Queen Bess—and me. The queen
bowed to sweep out a mess of Drano cans
from under the sink and a clink of glass
made her lean lower to see. Whiskey!
She snatched that bottle and slung it
from her hip through the open window
and the closed screen, and then went back to singing,
into a world of woe,

 as she scrubbed the sink clean. I never knew
my granddaddy. *We kept him away from you,*
Mama told me when I was older,
because he drank. Which explained Grandmother's
reaction. A Depression wife, she'd learned
to always save back a bit for leaner times,
so I guess she had saved a fat purse
of rage to spend that morning

on one mighty splurge of fury that ended
too fast to frighten me. It made me think,
though, and what I saved from that morning
was knowing when bad times came, I could fling
them out a window and keep on singing.
Years later, this saved me.

Losing

We are each other's memories. What I forget, you remember. And vice-versa.

—Sue Henry

Hymn

Only the living can sing,
but the dead can hear.

You are our voices,
they whisper,
but we are your ears.
Your songs can't be heard without us.

We who can sing owe a debt
to the dead.
Our notes are what's left
of their breath.
Our songs can't be voiced without them.

How can we use what was lost,
yet how can we not?

Their last exhalations
loft to our lungs
as gift or penance.
Their songs won't be sung without us.

When It Happened

It was one of those heavy July nights
when the day wouldn't let go its sweaty hug
on my old farm in north Georgia. A thrush
was chiming in the night with cool *pling, plinks*
like the water that drops from rocks in our creek,
but I was a mess of sweat and twigs
in the heart of our blueberry thicket,
my hair held fast by a blackberry cane.

Mama? Are you still there? I ripped free,
lowering myself like a flag so as not
to put out an eye on branches just
inches away, and I set down my pail. *Honey?*
Mama sounded calmly concerned. *I'm here,*
but I don't know what I can do to help.
Well, nothing, I guess. Still hunkered, I fell
to my knees and low-crawled through roots to where

I'd left her sitting picking the low berries
from her lawn chair, at least in theory.
She had gathered three cats and four berries
while I'd doggedly taken my chances
with snakes and poison ivy in quest of
the fattest fruit. *Do you need more?* She waved
a hand vaguely. More cats? Lord, no. She gave me
a look. No, Mama. I'll pick the rest.

She's eighty-nine, I reminded myself.
If she chooses not to pick, that's her right.
Honey, you do too much. Well, it's still light
and I wanted to finish before we left.
Left for where? I shoved Chloe over—*mrrupp*—

and perched on the porch of Daddy's old shop
to scratch the cat's calico head while I thought.
Was Mama kidding? We'd talked earlier--

no, actually, it was just before
I got stuck inside the blueberries. Ten
minutes ago? Maybe fifteen? I bent
to pick off a tic on Chloe's ear.
She bit me. Mama laughed: *Can you blame her? Sometimes
she gets tired of being messed with.* Thanks, Mom.
We're all going out; don't you remember?
Out? Out where? I don't want to. She stood up
and the flimsy chair went flying. I dove for
the chair, for her. *Who's going out? What for?*
And quit grabbing at me. Chloe left us;
cats hate a ruckus. For dinner, Mama.
All of us. It's my birthday. Her eyes flashed,
her green Irish eyes, a sign she was mad,
but too much of lady to let on.

Well, then, someone should have reminded me.
She strode back inside with her dignity
and Chloe, close after. Yep, she was mad,
not because I hadn't reminded her,
but because I had.

Placing the Blame

And so the angry years began.
Her world had tilted to one side
and maybe it was me whose hand
had tweaked its calibrations by
a smidge and tipped her world just out
of sync with what she'd always known
and trusted to be truth. To doubt
her own perceptions would have thrown
her to the wolves of helplessness,
and she was Irish independent.
Her other choice, a wilderness
of darkening cognition, meant
leaving us behind, and who
would she be then? It wasn't fair.
She'd saved me once, that much she knew.
So why was I not saving her?

Becoming a Traitor

Lord help me, I'm stealing my mother's mail.
What else can I do? She's sending money
to every so-called scam contest. *Honey,*
she smiles when I catch her, *It's okay. I'll*
get my money back. See? I'm already
a winner. Mama, they say you *may* be.
That's their loophole. *No, Honey, they called me.*
They have my name. Mama, they know you're ninety;
they've got your number. *That's what I just said.*
Why do you twist everything? Sheesh, I'm trying
to straighten things out. *Young Lady, listen*
to me. There's nothing wrong with my head.
I'll do what I want. You're doing what they
want. *They? Who are they?* I don't know. Do you?
I know the man who called me. His name is Dave.
No, it isn't. He made that up. *Can you*
prove it? No, Mama, I can't. *There you go.*
You have nothing to back up your claim, but I
have my name on this mail. It's my choice, my
mail.

    Not anymore. But she doesn't know.

I May Already Be a Winner

Hope comes in the mail six days a week.
Why does she hide it from me? Haven't I
always gotten by on hope and a deep,
abiding belief in goodness? I trust my
instincts, but apparently my daughter
doesn't. You can't send them money, *she says.*
Well, why not? Money's a fool's treasure.
When I was eight, money jumped from rooftops
over Wall Street and faded as it fell.
The year I turned eighteen, money grew cold
as steel for tanks, for guns, for planes, for shells,
for ships like the carrier that stole
my young husband and gave me back the man
I lived with the rest of his life. When
I was forty-eight, money from our friends
paid off her new patchwork of skin, and
this sneakiness is how she thanks them.
Honey, Honey—someone's mailing me hope.
It's worth the risk. Money slips from our hands
like memories. Let me choose to let it go.
I'm past caring where it lands.

Pills

It's their order that matters, not what the pills are for.
Why else would she get so upset if I take
them out of order? I've set a silver tray
to store the bottles on my drainboard;
the tray is small and round like a sliver clock
with amber bottles marking three and six
and nine and twelve. Each morning while I fix
my cereal, I take my pills. It works:
four bottles, four spots. There's thyroid at nine,
and heart at twelve, blood pressure at three.
The pill at six is to help me eat,
she says, but I'm dubious. I line
them up and start: Heart, twice a day.
Take one, take another. Done for today.

Equivocating

Who am I to say
my mama isn't right?
We've always come at life
so differently, this may
be like her cancelled checks,
from pre-Eisenhower up to
today at half-past two,
collated into stacks
of folders, labeled, stored
in hanging files, secured
against the day the world
might ask her for June fourth's
electric bill, nineteen-
sixty-two. *Here you go,*
she'd say. Whereas, I know
I pay my bills on time.
Can't they trust me on it?
If Mama says she's got
a system figured out
to help her not forget
to take her pills, I want
to trust her on it. It's my
concern, but it's her life.
I just need her to be right.

Ironing

It's peaceful and productive.
I can listen to my music
while I iron. The cats lie near
and nap.

Sometimes, I have to wait until
 my daughter comes to start the tape
machine. It isn't that I can't;
I won't.

I just have no desire to learn,
but she never minds about that.
I start singing and when she comes in,
she joins

her deeper alto to mine, or
sometimes she tries the soprano line
and mind you. the operative word
is tries.

I really don't give a hoot. Our singing
puts us together. She watches her pitch
and forgets to watch me. My
pitch holds.

I wish we'd forget the blessed tape
and just sing. I have a true ear;
she has a true heart. Sometimes, she
can't hear

what I'm trying to say, so her heart
works too hard. I hear her

gentling her words for me, and
it hurts

to know the way our places
have gotten so turned around, but
our singing is always easy. It's peaceful
and productive,

and the cats can curl up on the sofa
and nap.

Call and Response

How long has it been since you saw your doctor?
Lord, Honey, I don't know. I'm fine.
Do you want me to make an appointment for you?
I certainly don't. I can call him myself.

But you won't; you won't.

Sounds good. And I'll drive you there.
Oh, no you won't. I can still drive.
Come on, let me be your chauffeur.
You're busy. You don't need anything else.

You're right, I don't; I don't.

I'm fine. And I like your company.
I don't know why. I'm boring and old.
You've never been boring a day in your life.
Well, I bore myself. Give me the phone.

Which is your biggest fear?
Which do you not want to know?
Thank you, this means a lot to me.
I love you, too, but you're heartless and cold.
It's not like he's going to tell you you're dying.
Well, I never intended to live this long.

How can I keep her here?
How can I help her go?

Not to Complain, But

There ought to be a law against more than
two hospital stays per lifetime. Three, max.
And if one of those incarcerations
is for someone else's operation,
not my own, but I'm along for support,
I should instantly earn bonus points
and a free ride home.

In actuality, these partner stays
fall under a rider clause that relates
to restitution for my fourteenth year,
not to mention the travails of my birth.
Certain conditions apply. I qualify
for an orange fold-out sleeper chair that might
fold out or might not.

We both get a thousand-watt, room-wide
fluorescent fixture that stays on all night
because no one finds the remote until
the morning you leave. My signature will
be required for all choices I'd rather
not make, but I shouldn't expect any answers
to when and whether

and what if. Especially not what if.
We qualify for need-to-know status,
nothing more, and a tired and harried staff
will determine what we need to know. Last,
but not least for their purposes, we'll be
sent home with gibberish printouts I must keep
on file forever.

Cancer

You know when something's wrong inside of you,
at least, I do. I knew when I would lose
another baby, and when one finally stuck,
I knew that, too. I wouldn't take those drugs
to keep me from miscarrying. If it's not
meant to be, then there's a reason for it,
and best to let that baby go. Two, though,
I kept and carried home. With them, I knew.

So when the doctor said this mass was cancerous,
it wasn't news to me. I trust
the lady surgeon to do right by me;
she knows we're doing this for them, not me.
She'll clean out all of it, or else she won't,
and I can live with that until I don't.

There is a Fountain

Rage, rage against the dying of the light.
—Dylan Thomas

She woke so softly from her surgery,
as if on any morning. This is good,
I thought, and smiled with weary gratitude
at her, for her, for all of us, for me
and my unaltered life. *Did I die?*
She smiled at me and looked around. *If so,*
I don't approve of heaven. I said, no,
you'll see your surgeon soon. You did just fine.

I woke to someone ranting in our room:
Hello? I'll see my doctor now. Hello!
You saw her, Mama. What's the matter? *No!*
She's in the hall. She hears me. She won't come.
All night, my mama's mind lashed out and fought
with anesthesia's demons. And she lost.

Inoperable

Here tenderness and rage pace hand in hand
within this narrowed space where you and she
have found yourselves consigned unwillingly.
It's true, of course, that any place you stand
together is a home, but this one seems
to have no windows and its only door
leads in to stay, or so they say. No more
before, and after is a darkened room.

But now is yours, just as it always was,
and there's a steady generosity
inherent to each day with everything
you've known and shared still here and not yet lost
to future time's diminishing. Is this
a comfort? Yes. Is this a curse? It is.

The Lists

*Long-term cognitive disturbances are common
disabling consequences of anesthesia in the elderly.*
—British Journal of Anesthesia

It seemed the only way to save her life was by taking it away bit by
    bit,
but since it hurt to see her hands so empty, in place of choices we
    gave her lists:

Wednesday, March 22nd—Caregiver, ten-thirty to two-thirty,
    Meals on Wheels,
eye doctor appointment at three-thirty. And then two spaces to
    sign for her pills,

because she wouldn't believe us when we said she had taken her
    pills. She wanted
to believe herself, and that seemed fair. Morning and evening, she
    signed and handed

Mama's Daily Planner back to one of us. There, she'd say, with a
    look that let it
be known she had once again made her own choice to be in our
    debt.

Cats on the Hill

When my husband came home, his GI Bill paid
tuition and books and a little allotment
for food. His dad sent two hundred dollars that went
for the rest, and when I paid that back, I made
a note in the ledger I kept those early years.
But I'd forgotten how good I was until
she found the ledger:: Paid the power bill
on time, with four cents for savings left over.

I'm taking a count of the cats on the hill outside
my window today. Seven, but she says three,
and laughs. We laugh. I say, I'll try not to see
more cats, whether they're real or not, alright?
But in my head I make a note: four cats
left over for me, whether she sees them, or not.

Pitched Past Grief

—For Don

This is my hymn to weariness
after another night
not sleepless, but sleeping in fits between
rising to help her rise
and rising again to lay her down
between clean sheets.
We leave the piano lamp on
all night and lift the cat
from her feet in and out of the light
as we change the sheets--
a tabby cat, our hands. Her face
is soft with forgetfulness
that is the gift of sleep. Tired
beyond words, beyond
the fix of one good night of rest,
these holes in our nights
drain us during our days, but we've come
to love what is commonplace:
the jarring calls to help her rise,
this stuporous routine,
the lessening weight of her
leaning in and out of the light.

No

I did what I could until I can't.
Today, my hands, not on her skin
that needs to be washed clean. Not there.
Her face, her legs, her arms, her hands,
I can. But here what's asked of me
becomes the answer, no. If she
could own her words again, she'd say
it' s right to not feel right this way
about her waiting flesh and my
denying hands. She'd say that I
am hers, not she is mine. I should
back off while what I've done is good.

Keep on the Sonny Side

—For Sonny Houston, who is once again singing with Mama

Sonny's coming at two to sing with you,
I tell her after lunch. It's better not to
leave her too much time to fret or forget
or to look forward. Singing with Sonny lets
chaos take a break because music lives
under her daily weathers, deep-rooted.
Winter's coming on. Today I bundle
her in grey fleece as we wait for Sonny.
Lift your arms, Mama. She smiles and shrugs: *How?*
I raise the arms that raised me. Okay, now
let's move you to where you can see him play.
But one of her legs can't recall the way
to step and step again, so I sing,
Stand up, stand up for Jesus, ye soldiers,
until her legs obey the higher order
of music's steadfastness, so long as we
all keep singing.

Finding the Pattern

My daughter is standing
between the big window and me,
inside the sun and her hair. Honey,
your hair is absolutely beautiful.
What are you doing, Mama? *Well,*
I need to get these boxes lined up.
They have a pattern, but it's not right yet.
She sits to look and almost steps on one.
I pat her curls and the sun
spins in and out of my hands.
I made that hair. I made her. Look, Honey.
See those two there by your feet?
They keep moving. Something's not right.
I don't know, Mama. You'll figure it out.
My daughter's voice makes the boxes go still,
so I lie back and think.
She goes to the kitchen to get my dinner,
and the sun moves with her.

Aneurysm

They used to call pneumonia Old Man's Friend
because of how it shut a man's lungs against
the languid drift of prostate cancer's pain
relentlessly engulfing bone and brain.
An old man simply lost his breath, instead,
and died in days, not years. When Mama left her bed
without us seeing her, no one was near
enough to break her fall. We covered her,
a brittle heap of moaning, to keep her warm
and padded her hip, and waited for help to come,
but Mama's body had one kindness left
as thanks for all her years of tending it--
a clot broke from the cradle of her womb
and caught her like a hand to guide her home.

Elegy

Never to sing beside her again
is the gift and curse of her going.
Our altos clashed in life. Hers rang light
and pure, mine hangs low and dark as night.
We were the sun and moon of singing.
We always sang together facing
each other across a room, our tones
blending on music's sweet horizon
of harmonics where our voices
settled into sense, not discord. This
need to keep a distance for beauty's
sake died with her. Walking the woods with
my dogs, I sing wherever I please,
but her gone voice hums and haunts me.

Curriculum Vitae

Fate found us.
Fire proved us.
Pain bound us.
Life moved us.
Age caught you.
Need brought me.
Rage sought you.
Need taught me.
Love used me,
abused me.
Earth shook you.
Blood took you.

Loosed by your leaving.
Bound by my grieving.

Acknowledgements

The following poems appeared originally in *Alchemy*, a chapbook from Sow's Ear Press: *How it Happened, The Hardest Part, On My Other Hand, Some of Us*. Many thanks to Larry Richman for believing in me back then.

Boundless gratitude to the Hambidge Center for Arts and Sciences and to Everglades National Park for providing residencies during the writing of these poems.

Thank you to Linda Parsons for championing this book.

Thank you again to Larry Germain for always being willing to turn his musician's ear and editor's eye to my writing, and to the rest of my colleagues at the Wimberley Center, for being so endlessly supportive.

And to my family. Love always.